Keto 1
Weight

Text Copyright © 2018 Rick Elliott

Legal & Disclaimer

Legal & Disclaimer

The information contained in this book and its contents is not designed to replace or take the place of any form of medical or professional advice; and is not meant to replace the need for independent medical, financial, legal or other professional advice or services, as may be required. The content and information in this book has been provided for educational and entertainment purposes only.

The content and information contained in this book has been compiled from sources deemed reliable, and it is accurate to the best of the Author's knowledge, information and belief. However, the Author cannot guarantee its accuracy and validity and cannot be held liable for any errors and/or omissions. Further, changes are periodically made to this book as and when needed. Where appropriate and/or necessary, you must consult a professional (including but not limited to your doctor, attorney, financial advisor or such other professional advisor) before using any of the suggested remedies, techniques, or information in this book.

Upon using the contents and information contained in this book, you agree to hold harmless the Author from and against any damages, costs, and expenses, including any legal fees potentially resulting from the application of any of the information provided by this book. This disclaimer applies to any loss, damages or injury caused by the use and application, whether directly or indirectly, of any advice or information presented, whether for breach of contract, tort, negligence, personal injury, criminal intent, or under any other cause of action.

You agree to accept all risks of using the information presented inside this book.

You agree that by continuing to read this book, where appropriate and/or necessary, you shall consult a professional (including but not limited to your doctor, attorney, or financial advisor or such other advisor as needed) before using any of the suggested remedies, techniques, or information in this book.

Contents

Introduction

The Ketogenic diet has been considered as one of the hardest diets to follow. Counting calories and the need to include certain food preference in your meals may look daunting to some. It's probably the biggest reason many people turn their backs on it, even before getting started in earnest.

Many have this mindset that the Ketogenic diet is diet for the rich as they think of expensive foods like salmon, cheese, cheese, steak, bacon, etc. In some places, these foods are considered a luxury. People who try to get started with the diet, often end up getting back to carb-stuffed meals. " It's not sustainable for me. And I haven't lost weight yet!" as they are constrained by their budget.

But do you know that budget should never be an issue when it comes to the Keto Diet? There are myriad of ways you can achieve the same results even when you're on a tight budget.

In this book, we will reveal some of the many ways to take advantage of Ketogenic health benefits, even without spending much on your food and meals. It's just a matter of changing the way you think and the way you look at how Ketogenic meals. Provided are tips on how to simplify your meals and not go beyond your budget. Included are 30 Ketogenic recipes that are delightfully easy to prepare, and cheap!

Chapter 1: Go Simple on Your Keto

When budget tends to be of great concern, perhaps even hindering you from keeping with Ketogenic diet requirements. Going to a simple Ketogenic diet will do the trick.

In case you have forgotten how a Ketogenic diet works, you use up fat to fuel your body instead of the usual primary source, carbohydrates. You must see to it that your daily calorie intake consists of:

- 70% fat
- 25% calories
- 5% carbs

Our body is used to getting its energy from carbs because most of our meals are usually high in carb content. Only when your carb content is used up, will your body enter into ketosis - a state when the human body starts to draw its energy from stored fats.

By bringing down your carb content and increasing fat content in your food intake, your body will be forced to use your stored fat – the visceral fat on your belly. The visceral fat easily affects your vital organs as it surrounds your liver, pancreas, and intestines. Thus, having too much of the visceral fat can be harmful to your health.

While you continue with the Keto diet, your body will get used to using fat as the primary source of fuel, instead of carbs. Using up fats regularly will boost your energy and metabolism and keep your body from gaining visceral fat.

An average man needs to have a daily intake of 2,500 calories and 2,000 for women. So based on this, you should limit your calories to:

For Men (2,500 calories)
Fats (70%): 1,750 calories/194 grams
Protein   (25%): 625 calories/ 156 grams
Carbohydrates   (5%): 125 calories/ 31 grams

For Women (2,000 calories)
Fats (70%): 1,400 calories/ 156 grams
Protein   (25%): 500 calories/ 125 grams
Carbohydrates   (5%): 100 calories/ 25 grams

- There are 9 calories in every gram of fat
- There are 5 calories in every gram of protein

- There are 5 calories in every gram of carbohydrates

Sticking to this basic nutrition principle of Keto, it's perfectly alright to eat food you love eating.

However, a typical diet is 35% fat, 15% protein, and 59% carbohydrates. When you start calorie counting and note how much you are taking of this and that, that's when the Keto diet gets intimidating to most people. When you start to worry about what you'll eat for your next meal, you consciously start avoiding the diet. You may have tried getting started but stopped as soon as you get tired of counting those macros. But a Keto diet could be easy and doesn't take much of your mental energy if you can follow these simple rules.

Rule # 1 - Limit Carbs

Many find this rule hard to follow. With Keto, you can't have foods that contain more carbohydrates than what you actually need. With vegetables and avocado, you can have 25 grams of carbs and 14 grams

Rule #2 - Start your Day with a Fat-Filled Breakfast

You need your energy for the rest of the day and your goal is to get about a third of your fat requirement for starters. Most people fail at Keto because they tried to skip breakfast as they rush to work. A cup of Keto coffee is about 14 grams of fat and a usual meal contains less than 25 grams of fat. Even when you have 50-75 grams of fat for two meals and 2 cups of coffee, you are a long way to filling up your daily fat requirement of 156-194 grams of fats.

At night, when you are less active, you don't burn as much fat as you do in the morning. Fat intakes that aren't used up are stored as visceral fat.

When most people fail to take their breakfast or earlier meal, they often end up loading on their dinner as they reach the end of the day.

Now that you know the effect of loading too much fat at night, it is best that you load your breakfast with fat instead, so you don't end up cramming too much fat at the end of the day. If you have 3 eggs in your breakfast plate (15 grams), 4 bacon slices (15 grams), and a cup of Keto coffee (14 grams), that would add up to 44 grams of fat before starting the day!

Rule#3 – Load your Meals with Fats

Every time you are preparing your meals, remember to have more fat than protein and carbs combined. Make sure you are taking in good fats and not the bad fat. When the issue of budgeting comes in, remember that there are always cheaper options for every expensive food item on your list.

Rule #4 – Track and Adjust

The first three rules are simple but while you are adjusting to it, it's best to keep track and do some adjustment to ensure success. The easiest way to track your performance is through your weight. If you can see changes in your weight, like weight loss, then you're on the right track.

Another way is through urine testing. There are ketone pee strips available in the market which you can use. These ketone strips will instantly let you know if your body is producing ketones, especially during your first two weeks after getting started.

Another method is testing through blood. There is a device that will allow you to analyze through your blood sample whether you are in a ketosis or not.

Any of the above tests will give you an overview of how well you are doing with the Keto diet. However, when you think that your diet isn't working based on your test results, here are three ways to correct.

Make sure your carbs are within keto limits – no sweeteners and starchy foods. Even fruits have carbs, so make sure to include them in your counting.

Reduce meat and high-protein food intake. When you are taking more protein than what your body actually needs, amino acids present in protein will be converted into glucose and can eventually damage your kidney. This can pose a problem especially when you're on the Keto diet as it prevents your body from undergoing complete ketosis.

Reduce your total food intake. When you aren't losing weight despite following keto rules, you're probably overeating. Cut your food quantity by simply eating less than what you're used to. It will be hard to adjust initially, but as your body adapts to the Keto diet, you'll be surprised to find it easy to live on.

Chapter 2: Keto Budgeting Guide

To some people, Keto foods are usually a luxury. It's however, not impossible to eat quality Keto meals on a budget. Careful planning and seeing what available resources you have, makes this possible. With a little adjustment, you may even be able to save some money compared to when you are eating those expensive high-carb diets.

You can start by making an inventory and evaluation of your pantry. If you want to save money, one thing you should consider is the food wastage. Make sure you don't buy stocks you won't be able to consume within its life shelf.

In addition to that, here are some tips to consider so you maximize on the benefits of ketogenic diet at minimal cost.

Buy in Bulk

It's practical and cost-efficient to buy food in bulk. Aside from the time and money you spent going to and fro to buy them, buying food on wholesale prices is relatively cheaper than getting them at a retail cost.

Buy only what is needed. You may do your marketing once a week, so make a list of what you can consume in a week's time. Here is when planning and preparing your Ketogenic budget menu matters. You can make an estimate of what to buy and how many of each item you're going to need. You don't want to buy more than you need and end up spoiling them or keeping them in the fridge without knowing if they are still suitable for use.

Planning

Plan meals you are going to prepare for the week. It wouldn't take much time to sit down and take a few hours to prepare a weekly meal plan. From there, you will be able to see what you want to achieve out of your Keto diet and how you want it done.

Begin by searching for recipes that are suitable to both your taste buds and pocket-friendly!

- Meals to prepare - Breakfast, lunch, snacks, and dinner.

- Shopping list – List down what you need so you can avoid buying on impulse. You can also save time if you stick to your list.

- Shopping schedule - How often would you go shopping? It's best to replenish your pantry every week.

Cook in Bulk

If you can buy in bulk, then you might as well cook in bulk. For example, if you have more mouths to feed or when you don't have too much time to spend in the kitchen. Meal prep is simply preparing your meals ahead by cooking in bulk and dividing into portions allocated within 5-7 days. Meal Prep saves you time on shopping and cooking.

Buy in Season

When buying fruits and vegetables, choose those that are in season for they are likely to be cheaper. Remember the Law of Demand and Supply? When there's more supply of those items, competition is high and prices of these products will be lower.

Buy Food at Nearest Location

It's always convenient to go online shopping, especially for your meal preparation. Aside from getting the best prices from among competitive sources, you can do your shopping in between work hours or while relaxing at home.

Because competition is tough in online shopping, suppliers go all out to provide shoppers with the best deals and user experience. Discounts, coupons, promotional items, and many more. Take advantage of these and you can save more.

Regardless of perks, when shopping online, you have to primarily consider the location of these suppliers. Choose ones that are nearest to you to save on shipping cost.

Chapter 3: Budget Shopping List

Meats

In Keto diet, you don't always have to include meats in every meal. Too much protein-based food will kick you out of ketosis. However, when you need to have meat, beef, pork, and chicken are commonly used. Also, choice cuts like thighs and breasts are popular among recipes; buying whole chicken is less-expensive and could save you a lot on your budget.

Minced Beef - this can be used for egg rolls and bun-less burgers.

Sausages - Read labels carefully for carb content

Eggs and Dairy

Eggs are all the same as long as you choose the organic ones. Although some are more expensive than others depending on where they come from or where you are buying. Eggs sold in the market is cheaper since most come from local suppliers.

Dairy (cheese, butter, cream, and sour cream)

Vegetables

Never neglect vegetables especially when you are thinking of your budget. Choosing veggies with low carb counts can provide you with more fibers and other nutrients essential to your health. Ideally, half of your meals should consist of greens.

Zucchini, Brussels sprouts cauliflower, cabbage - there are too many recipes using these vegetables and they are always in season. You can buy them anytime and create a variety of meals using them.

Fruits

Avocado is a must when considering acceptable food in the Keto diet. It contains 2 net carbs per 100 grams and a rich source of iron, zinc, magnesium, and manganese.

Spices and seasonings

They are much cheaper when fresh and if you want to save more, you can even try drying some of the herbs so you don't have to buy those expensive herbs and spices on bottles.

Chapter 4: 30 Cheap and Easy Recipes

#1 - Cabbage Rolls

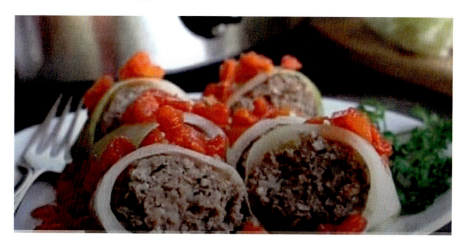

Ingredients

- 1 Head of cabbage

- 1 lb. Ground meat

- 15 oz. Tomatoes (diced)

- 2 cups Cauliflower rice

- 1 small Onion (diced)

- 2 tsp. Italian seasoning

- ½ tsp. Pepper

- 2 Cloves of Garlic

- 1 tsp. Salt

Directions

1. In a large mixing bowl, combine all the ingredients excluding the cabbage.

2. Lay cabbage leaves, one at a time on a large plate.

3. Fill up each leaf with the meat-cauliflower mixture (about ¼ cup). Roll it like a burrito.

4. Cover the inner bottom of a slow cooker with a thin layer of diced tomatoes, evenly spread.

5. Place the cabbage roll with its seam facing down over diced tomatoes.

6. Top it with remaining diced tomatoes and cook at high heat for 2-3 hours. When you opt to cook at low heat, cook for 4-6 hours.

7. Serve and enjoy!

Nutritional Value: Calories –120; Net Carbs – 8 grams; Protein – 5 grams; Fat – 4 grams

#2 – Cauliflower Hash Browns

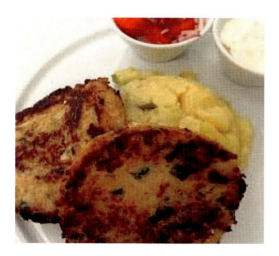

Ingredients

- 3 Large eggs

- ½ Yellow onions (grated)

- 15 oz. Cauliflower

- 4 oz. Butter

- Salt and pepper to taste

Directions

1. Cleanse and trim your cauliflowers and grind in a food processor.

2. Transfer the processed cauliflower in a mixing bowl and add remaining ingredients. Toss to blend and set aside for later use.

3. In a large skillet, melt the butter over medium heat.

4. Place about 3 scoops of the cauliflower mixture into the frying pan and flatten it to form a pancake. Fry the pancake until it turns light brown. Flip

to cook evenly on both sides. Adjust heat while cooking to prevent burning.

5.   Repeat the process until the batter is used up.

6.   Place cooked cauliflower hash browns on a plate and serve with leafy green salad.

Nutritional Value: Calories – 164; Net Carbs – 3 grams; Protein – 7 grams; Fat – 11 grams

#3 - Cauliflower Fried Rice

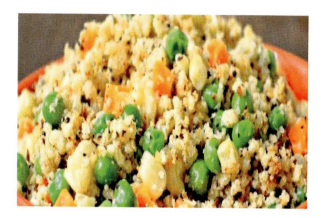

Ingredients

- 1 large head of cauliflower (chopped)
- ½ Shallots (minced)
- 1 Clove of garlic
- ½ cup Frozen corn (thawed)
- ½ cup peas and carrots (thawed)
- 2 tbsp. Soy sauce
- 2 tbsp. Olive oil

Directions

- Cleanse the cauliflower and cut into small florets. Using a food processor, pulse florets until it resembles the rice and set aside.

- Transfer the cauliflower florets to a bowl and add shallots, garlic with the blend of sesame oil.

- Preheat oven at 375 degrees Fahrenheit.

- Take a large baking dish and transfer the blended mixture into it. Spread evenly and roast the dish for about 8 minutes. Toss and spread again. Roast it for another 8 minutes for even cooking.

- Add vegetables to the cauliflower rice and roast for a couple of minutes more before pouring soy sauce on the mixture. Serve it with 2 scrambled eggs, chicken or shrimps.

Notes

You can easily sauté the cauliflower rice in a large skillet with onions and garlic. Add the rest of the ingredients when the onions become translucent.

Nutritional Value: Calories – 140; Net Carbs – 11 grams; Protein – 3 grams; Fat – 9 grams

#4 – Cauliflower Rice with Broccoli and Cheese

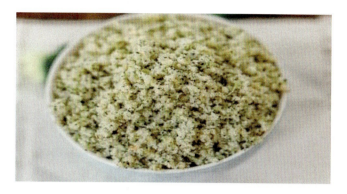

Ingredients

- 1 Large head of cauliflower

- 1 Broccoli (small)

- ½ cup shredded cheese

- 2 cups Cream cheese

- 1 tsp. Garlic powder

- 2 tbsp. Olive oil

- Salt and pepper to taste

Directions

1. Cleanse and cut cauliflower and broccoli into florets and run through a food processor until they are as fine as rice.

2. Place the mixture in a mixing bowl and add salt and pepper with olive oil. Mix to completely blend before transferring it to a large pan, spread evenly.

3. Preheat the oven to 350 degrees Fahrenheit and bake the dish for 10 minutes. Remove from the oven and mix. Again, spread it evenly on the pan and return it to the oven. Bake for another 10 minutes until. Add cream cheese and shredded cheese. Do the same process all over again until the cauliflower rice with broccoli turns golden brown in color. Serve and enjoy!

Nutritional Value: Calories – 96; Net Carbs – 4.7 grams; Protein – 4.1 grams; Fat – 6.4 grams

#5 - Crack Slaw

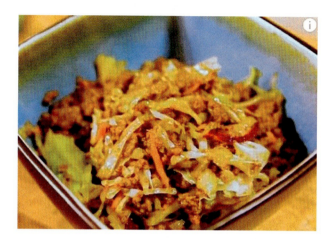

Ingredients

- 5 oz. Butter

- 20 oz. Ground beef

- 25 oz. Green cabbage

- 1 tsp. onion powder

- 2 Garlic Cloves

- 1 tsp. chili flakes

- 1 tbsp. Sesame oil

- 1 tbsp. Fresh ginger (grated or finely chopped)

- 3 Scallions (sliced)

- 1 tbsp. White wine vinegar

- 1/4 tsp. Ground black pepper

- 1 tsp. Salt

For Wasabi Mayonnaise

- 1/2 tbsp. wasabi paste
- 1 cup Mayonnaise

Directions

1. Dump cabbage in a food processor to process it into fine cuts.

2. Fry cabbage with about 2 0z of butter in a large frying pan at medium-high heat. Make sure you don't cook look enough for the cabbage to wilt or turn brown.

3. Droop spices and vinegar on the pan and continue to stir-fry for 2 minutes more. Transfer the cabbage to a bowl.

4. Melt the remaining butter using the same pan and sauté chili flakes, garlic, and ginger.

5. Add the meat and allow it to be thoroughly cooked until a little amount of the juice is left with the meat. Reduce heat to low and add cabbage and scallions. Stir and season with salt and pepper. Top the dish with sesame oil to serve.

6. Prepare the wasabi dressing by mixing Wasabi paste with Mayonnaise. The wasabi shall serve as the base so add mayonnaise little by little as you adjust the flavor. Sever stir-fry with wasabi dressing.

Nutritional Value: Calories – 164; Net Carbs – 6 grams; Protein – 8.5 grams; Fat – 12.3 grams

#6 – Cheese Roll-Ups

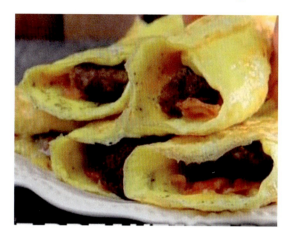

Ingredients

- 8 oz. Cheddar cheese (in slices)

- 2 oz. of butter

Directions

1. Lay slices of cheese on a large plate.

2. Slice butter thinly. You may use a cheese slicer for cutting.

3. Place butter slices on top of each slice of cheese and roll. Serve as a snack.

Note: You may add an extra taste by topping your butter with finely chopped parsley or any fresh herbs.

Nutritional Value: Calories – 466; Net Carbs – 76 grams; Protein – 37 grams; Fat – 30grams

#7 - Chicken Breast – Keto Recipe

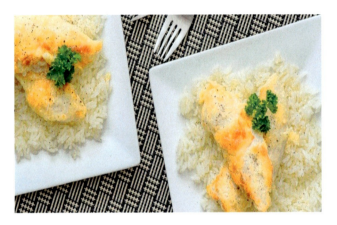

Ingredients

- ½ cup Parmesan cheese

- 5-6 Pcs Chicken breasts skinless and boneless)

- 1 cup Mayonnaise

- ½ tsp. Garlic powder

Directions

1. Mix all ingredients in a bowl including chicken breasts. Coat evenly on all sides

2. Arrange chicken breasts in single layer on a baking pan sprayed with oil.

3. Bake in the oven for 30-25 minutes at 375 degrees Fahrenheit.

Nutritional Value: Calories – 302.9; Net Carbs – 0 grams; Protein – 13.1 grams; Fat – 16.4 grams

#8 - Chicken Zoodle Soup

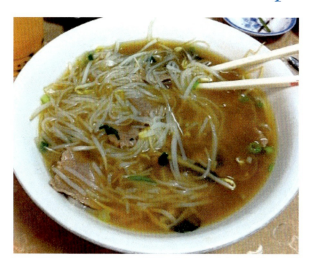

Ingredients

- 3 pcs. Medium-sized zucchini (spiraled)

- 2 tbs. Olive oil

- 1 lb. Chicken breasts (skinless, deboned, and cut into chunks)

- 3 carrots (diced)

- 3 Cloves of garlic (minced)

- 1 Onion (diced_

- 2 Celery stalks (sliced)

- Freshly ground black pepper

- 4 cups Chicken stock

- 2 tbsp. Lemon juice extract

- ¼ tsp. Dried rosemary

- 1 Bay leaf

- ½ tsp. Dried thyme

- 2 tbsp. Fresh parsley leaves (chopped)

- 1 sprig of fresh rosemary

Directions

1. Pour a tablespoon of olive oil in a large stockpot. Heat it over medium heat.

2. In a mixing bowl, season chicken with salt and pepper and transfer it to the stockpot. Allow it to cook until it turns golden brown and then set aside.

3. Pour remaining oil into the pot and sauté carrots and celery with garlic and onions. Cook until the carrots are tender before stirring in thyme and rosemary for about an hour.

4. Add chicken stock with 2 cups of water along with the bay leaf. Bring to a boil and stir in chicken and zucchini noodles. Allow it to simmer by reducing heat until zucchini becomes tender. This takes about 3 minutes. Add lemon extract and season with salt and pepper.

5. Serve while warm and garnish with fresh parsley and rosemary.

Nutritional Value: Calories – 317; Net Carbs – 28 grams; Protein – 42 grams; Fat – 7 grams

#9 - Cobb Egg Salad

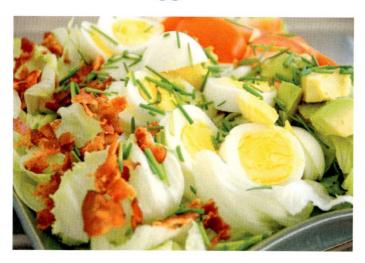

Ingredients

- 6 Large eggs (hard boiled)

- ¼ cup Blue cheese (crumbled)

- ¼ cup Arugula

- 6 tbsp. Mayonnaise

- 2 tsp. Dry Ranch dressing mix

- ¼ cup Cheddar cheese (finely shredded)

- 4 Bacon (fried and chopped)

- ¼ cup Grape tomatoes (diced)

Directions

1. Peel eggs and chopped. Place in a large mixing bowl and combine the rest of the ingredients. Toss to blend.

2. Serve in a sandwich or with crackers.

Nutritional Value: Calories – 115; Net Carbs – 2.9 grams; Protein – 6.4 grams; Fat – 8.6 grams

#10 - Crockpot Cabbage Rolls

Ingredients

- 1 Head of cabbage

- 1 lb. Meat (ground)

- 1 Small onion (diced)

- 2 tbsp. Italian seasoning

- 15 oz. Tomatoes (diced)

- 2 cups Cauliflower rice

- 1 1/2 tsp. Salt

- 2 Cloves of garlic (minced)

- 1/2 tsp. Pepper

Directions

1. Combine the ground meat, cauliflower rice, garlic, and seasonings in a large mixing bowl. Add salt and pepper to taste.
2. Blanch cabbage leaf in boiling water for about 5 minutes then have it run under cool water.
3. Lay a leaf of the cabbage on a plate or flat surface.
4. Take about 2 spoonful of the meat mixture and fill up each leaf.
5. Roll to wrap like in a burrito.
6. cover the bottom of the crockpot with diced tomatoes
7. Put the cabbage rolls on top of the tomatoes with seam-side down.
8. Pour over the rolls the remaining diced tomatoes and cook high for 2-3 hours.

Nutritional Value: Calories – 152; Net Carbs – 3.9 grams; Protein – 19.5 grams; Fat – 2.6grams

#11 - Cream Cheese Pancake

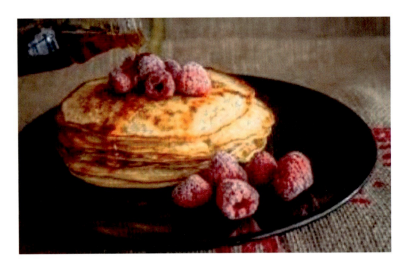

Ingredients

- 2 Large Eggs

- 1/2 tsp. Cinnamon

- 1 tsp. Granulated sugar substitute

- 2 oz. Cream Cheese

Directions

1. Add all the ingredients to a blender or food processor and process until smooth in its consistency

2. Stop for a while to allow bubbles to settle.

3. Prepare a pan sprayed with cooking oil. Place into the pan about 1/4 of the batter. Cook for about 2 minutes over medium-high heat until it turns golden brown. Flip and cook for another minute for even cooking.

4. Cook remaining batter in batches until fully used up.

5. Serve with sugar-free syrup along with berries or any fruit of your choice.

Nutritional Value: Calories –344; Net Carbs – 2.5 grams; Protein – 17 grams; Fat – 29 grams

#12 - Creamy Tomato Soup

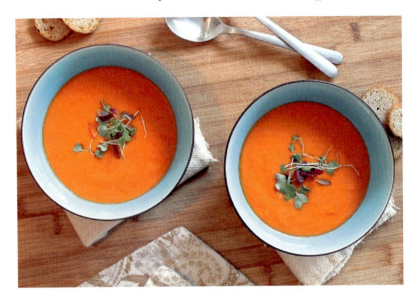

Ingredients

- 1 Clove of garlic

- 2 tbsp. Unsalted butter

- 2 14-oz. cans of Whole peeled tomatoes

- Freshly ground pepper (coarse)

- 1/2 Heavy cream

- 1 1/2 cups Chicken stock or plain water

- Salt to taste

Directions

1. Melt butter in a stockpot over medium heat and sauté garlic first and followed by onions. Stir constantly to prevent from burning until onions become translucent. This will take about 3 minutes.

2. Gradually add tomatoes including its juice and stock. Add salt and pepper to taste and let it boil. Once it reaches the boiling point, reduce heat and allow simmering for about 10 minutes.

3. Pour the tomato mixture into a food processor and puree.

4. Clean the pot and transfer back into it the tomato mixture. Cook over low heat. Add the cream and stir to combine. Serve warm.

Nutritional Value: Calories – 100; Net Carbs – 16 grams; Protein – 5 grams; Fat – 2 grams

#13 – Fried Cabbage

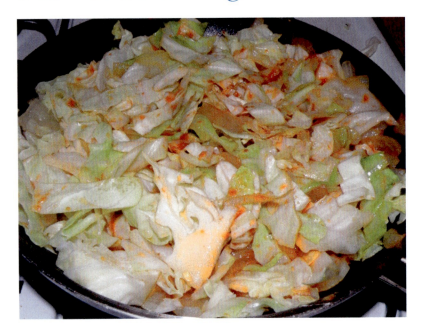

Ingredients

- 6 cups of cabbage (julienned)

- 3 Bacon sliced (chopped to pieces)

- 1 tbsp. Cider vinegar

- 2 tbsp. Water

- Salt and pepper to taste

Directions

1. Preheat a large deep skillet over medium to high heat. Roast bacon until evenly brown. Remove and set aside for later use.

2.   Sauté the onion until it becomes translucent and add the cabbage. Pour water and season with salt and pepper. Cook for about 15 minutes before adding in the bacon. Drizzle with vinegar before serving in a plate.

Nutritional Value: Calories – 47; Net Carbs – 2.8 grams; Protein – 5 grams; Fat – 5.2grams

#14 - Herb-Roasted Pork Loin

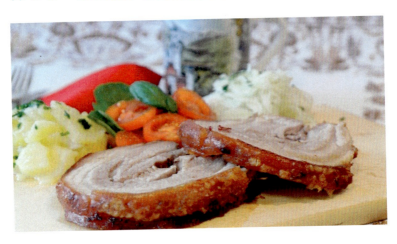

Ingredients

- 1 1/2 Pork loin

- 1 tsp. Dried basil

- 2 cloves of garlic (minced)

- 1 tsp. Dried rosemary

- 10 Fresh crack pepper

- 2 tbsp. Olive oil

- Salt to taste

Directions

1. Start by preheating the oven to 425 degrees Fahrenheit. Add seasonings, herbs, and spices in a food processor and pulse. Transfer the mixture to a mixing bowl and add oil. Toss to blend.

2. Prepare a baking pan or baking sheet. Align it with aluminum foil.

3. Rub and coat the pork with the mixture evenly on all sides. Arrange the pork in the baking pan in single layer and roast for about 45 minutes and until the pork is thoroughly cooked and browned. Wait for 10 minutes before taking the dish out of the oven.

4. Once ready, serve on a platter and garnish with the desired garnishing.

Nutritional Value: Calories – 148; Net Carbs – 1 gram; Protein – 25 grams; Fat – 8 grams

#15 - Lettuce-Wrapped Burger

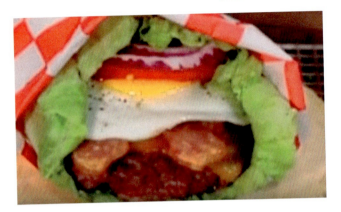

Ingredients

- 6 slices of American cheese

- 2 tomatoes, (in thin slices)

- 2 lbs. Lean ground beef

- 2 large heads of Romaine lettuce (cleaned and dried)

- 1 small Red onion (diced)

- 1 tsp. Dried oregano

- 1 tsp. Black pepper

- 1/2 tsp. Sea salt

Spread

- 1 tbsp. Dill pickle relish

- 3 tbsp. Ketchup

- ½ cup Light mayonnaise

- Salt and pepper to taste

Instructions

1. Preheat a skillet over medium heat.

2. Combine ground beef and oregano in a large mixing bowl. Season with salt and pepper.

3. Divide the beef mixture into 6 parts and have each part rolled into a ball. Using your palm, flatten balls to form patties.

4. Once the skillet is ready, cook patties but make sure they are not overcrowded. Cook until patties turn golden brown in color. Cook evenly on each side

5. While waiting for patties, prepare the spread. Add all spread ingredients in a mixing bowl and toss to blend. Chill in the fridge for later use.

6. Lay a large lettuce leaf on a large plate and place the onion over it. Top with a slice of cheese spread, a slice of tomato, onions or bell pepper).

Nutritional Value: Calories – 206; Net Carbs – 6 grams; Protein – 10 grams; Fat – 41 grams

#16 - Limed Chicken Drumsticks with Cilantro

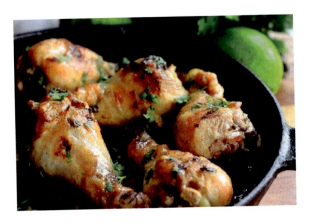

Ingredients

- 4 Cloves of garlic

- 2 tbsp. Olive oil

- 1/2 bunch of cilantro

- Freshly cracked pepper

- 1/2 tsp. cumin

- 2 Limes

- 6 Chicken drumsticks

- 1/2 tsp. salt

Directions

1. Add garlic, olive oil, cracked pepper, cumin and salt in a mixing bowl. Mix thoroughly. Likewise, add 2 tablespoon lime juice and a teaspoon lime to

the marinade mixture. Get some cilantro leaves and chop finely and sprinkle over the mixture. The remaining cilantro will be used after baking.

2. Pour marinade into a zip-lock bag along with chicken drumsticks. Securely close the bag and massage the content to coat the drumsticks evenly with the marinade. Refrigerate for 30 minutes or more while occasionally turning the bag.

3. Preheat oven to 400 degrees Fahrenheit and arrange drumsticks to a casserole dish in a single layer. Cook in batches if there are more but never overcrowded. Pour some marinade over the chicken drumsticks.

4. Bake for 45 minutes until browned, basting once in a while.

5. Once done, serve on a platter with fresh slices of lime and sprinkled finely-chopped cilantro leaves.

Nutritional Value: Calories – 46; Net Carbs – 1.6 grams; Protein – 0.18 grams; Fat – 4.6 grams

#17 - Low-Carb Cabbage Rolls

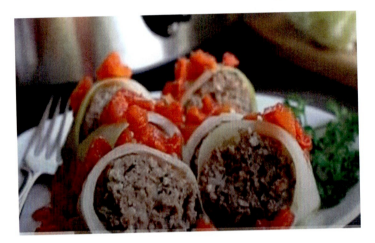

Ingredients

- 1 lb. Cabbage head

- 1/4 cup Parsley

- 1/2 lb. Ground beef

- 1 onion

- 2 cups Cauliflower (finely chopped)

- 1 Egg

- Salt and pepper to taste

Sauce

- 1/4 cup Sour cream

- A pinch of ground cloves

- 1 cup Tomato sauce

- Stevia to taste

Directions

1. Cleanse and core the cabbage.

2. Boil the water in a large pot (about 2-inch deep).

3. Steam cabbage until it becomes tender but still firm. Set aside.

4. Add cauliflower in a food processor and pulse to produce fine grains.

5. Cook beef with onion and drain. Place on a mixing bowl and combine with raw cauliflower and parsley. Season it with salt and pepper to taste.

6. Beat in egg and blend.

7. Lay a cabbage leaf on a flat surface and add about a tablespoon or two of the mixture. Roll up. Repeat the process until the mixture is used up.

Sauce

1. In a mixing bowl, add cloves, tomato, sour cream and sweetener to taste. Whisk until smooth.

2. If you want your sauce thin, just add a bit of water.

To Cook

1. Fill slow cooker with about 1/4 cup of water.

2. Lay rolls inside the cooker and pours over it the remaining sauce.

3. Cook for 6 hours. If you want less cooking time, bake in the oven at 350 degrees Fahrenheit for an hour. Serve.

Nutritional Value: Calories – 140; Net Carbs – 13 grams; Protein – 12 grams; Fat – 4 grams

#18 – Mushroom and Cheese Frittata

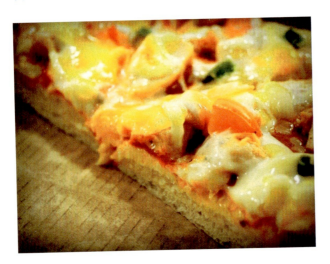

Ingredients

- Frittata

- 1 cup Mayonnaise

- 10 Large eggs

- 8 oz. Cheese (shredded)

- ½ tsp. Ground black pepper

- 4 oz. Leafy green

- 1 tbsp. Fresh parsley

- 15 oz. Mushrooms

- 6 Scallions

- 3 oz. Butter

Vinaigrette

- 1 tbsp. White wine vinegar

- 4 tbsp. Olive oil

- ¼ tsp. Ground black pepper

- 1 tsp. Salt

Directions

1. Start by preheating the oven to 350 degrees Fahrenheit. Proceed to prepare the vinaigrette and set aside for later use.

2. Slice mushroom into desired cuts.

3. Fried mushroom in a skillet over medium-high heat, using most of the butter. Lower heat and reserve remaining butter to grease the baking pan.

4. Chop scallions and add them to fried mushrooms. Mix in the parsley and season with salt and pepper to taste.

5. In a medium-size mixing bowl, add eggs and beat. Then add mayonnaise and cheese and make another round of beating to blend ingredients. Also, add the scallions and mushrooms. For the final touch, add salt and pepper to the egg mixture.

6. Pour the mixture into a well-greased pan and bake for 40 minutes. As soon as the Frittata turns golden brown, turn off the oven and allow it to cool down for about five minutes before serving. Serve with vinaigrette and leafy green veggies.

Nutritional Value: Calories – 180; Net Carbs – 5 grams; Protein – 18 grams; Fat – 10 grams

#19 – Omelette Waffle

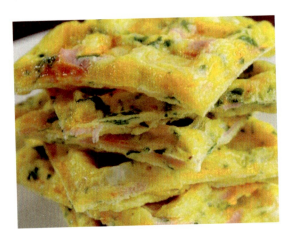

Ingredients:

- 1 tbsp. of Mozzarella cheese (shredded)

- 1 tbsp. Red pepper (finely chopped)

- 1 tbsp. Broccoli (finely chopped)

- 1 tbsp. of sausage (finely sliced)

- 2 tsp. Palm oil

Directions

1. Preheat waffle iron and spray with palm oil on both sides (top and bottom). In a mixing bowl, combine milk and egg and whisk to form the batter. Once the waffle molder is hot, pour the batter carefully. See to it that it is filled up just below the top level. Leave enough space to allow the waffle to rise. Filling up all the space will cause a leak on the sides, messing up your dish.

2. Cook in the same process until all batter is used up.

Nutritional Value: Calories – 317; Net Carbs – 1.63 grams; Protein – 7.67 grams; Fat – 30.92 grams

#20 - Pepperoni-Avocado Salad

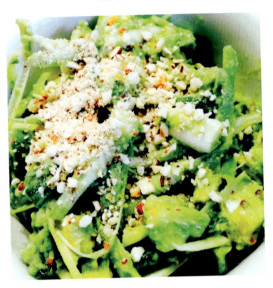

Ingredients

- 1 Avocado (cubed)

- Slices of Pepperoni

- 1 oz. Mozzarella pearls

- Italian seasoning or lime juice

- Salt and pepper

Directions

1. Combine all ingredients in the mixing bowl. Toss to blend and serve as appetizer or side dish.

Nutritional Value: Calories – 152; Net Carbs – 45/2 grams; Protein – 19.5 grams; Fat – 2.6 grams

#21 - Pork - Pineapple Kebabs

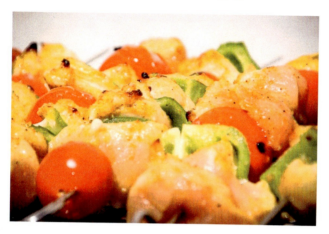

Ingredients

Marinade

- 1-inch Ginger (fresh and grated)

- 2 Cloves of garlic (minced)

- 1 tbsp. Honey

- 2 tbsp. Olive oil

- 2 tbsp. Soy sauce

Kebabs

- 1 tbsp. Vegetable oil

- 1 lb. Pork Chops (bones)

- 1 Onion

- 20-oz. can of Pineapple chunks (with juice)

- Salt and pepper to taste

For Garnishing

- Sriracha to taste

- One bunch of cilantro

Directions

- Cleanse skewers. If using bamboo materials, soak in water for about 30 minutes to keep it from burning.

- Prepare the marinade mixture by mixing garlic, ginger, oil, honey and soy sauce in a mixing bowl.

- Cut pork into desired slices. Marinate the pork in the marinade and chill in the fridge for 30 minutes.

- Drain juice from pineapple chunks. Cut bell peppers and onion by an inch and place them in a bowl. Add a tablespoon of oil and sprinkle with salt and pepper. Toss to coat evenly.

- Thread marinated skewers followed by either pineapple or onion and alternating bell pepper. Repeat the same process with the rest of the skewers until all are used up.

- Preheat the oven. Arrange the skewers on top of the rack placed over the pan. Cook for 5 minutes until edges starts to turn brown. Rotate the skewers and cook for another 5 minutes. Continue rotating until all sides are evenly browned and cooked.

- Serve kebabs with a squirt of Sriracha and garnish with freshly chopped cilantro.

Nutritional Value: Calories – 248; Net Carbs – 25.5 grams; Protein – 25.9 grams; Fat – 5 grams

#22 - Quinoa Tabbouleh

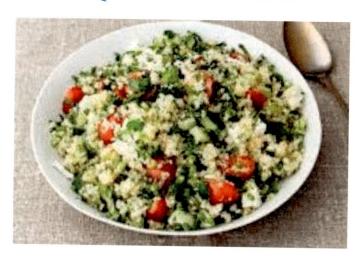

Ingredients

- 1/4 cup Olive oil

- 1 cup Quinoa rice (uncooked)

- 4 cloves of garlic

- 1 large lemon

- 1 Large cucumber

- A bunch of parsley

- 1 Large tomato

- 1 tsp. Salt

Directions

1. Cleanse and rinse quinoa rice and place it in a large pot filled with 1 3/4 cup water. Cover the pot and bring to boil over high heat. As it reaches the boiling point, lower down heat to allow simmering for 15 minutes.

After the allotted time, turn off the stove. Set aside to cool down before preparing the salad.

2. While waiting for quinoa to cool, make the dressing. In a large mixing bowl, squeeze the lemon to extract the juice. Add minced garlic and olive oil with salt. Toss to blend and set aside the dressing.

3. Cleanse all vegetables in water especially the parsley to remove sand. Start cutting tomatoes and cucumber into dice size. Also, cut parley finely. Combine tomato, parsley, and cucumber on a large mixing bowl.

4. Add the cooled quinoa along with vegetables. Pour dressing on top and make sure everything is coated. Serve quickly or chill in the before serving, give the salad a final stir.

Nutritional Value: Calories – 250; Net Carbs – 11 grams; Protein – 6 grams; Fat – 15 grams

#23 - Roasted Brussels Sprouts

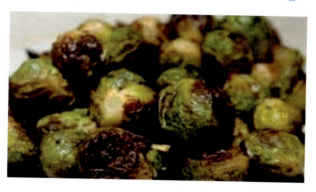

Ingredients

- 1.5 lbs. Brussels Sprouts (trimmed)

- 3 tbsp. Olive oil

Directions

1. Cleanse and trim Brussels sprouts and place in a large resealable plastic bag. Add olive oil and season with kosher salt and pepper. Seal the bag and shake to allow sprouts to be evenly coated.
2. Transfer to the baking pan and place inside the oven preheated at 200 degrees Fahrenheit.
3. Roast for 30 minutes but make sure to shake the pan every 5 minutes for even browning. Set to reduce heat to prevent burning. When it's almost black, take it out of the oven and serve.

Nutritional Value: Calories – 104; Net Carbs – 10 grams; Protein – 2.9 grams; Fat – 7.3 grams

#24– Roasted Garlic Lemon Broccoli

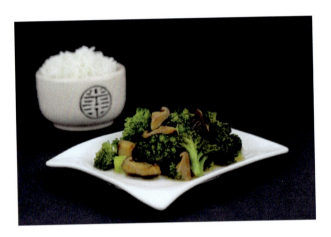

Ingredients

- 2 Broccoli heads (cut into florets)

- ½ tsp. Lemon extract

- 1 Clove of garlic

- 2 tsp. Extra-virgin Olive oil

- 1 tsp. Sea salt

- ½ tsp. Ground black pepper

Directions

1. Prepare oven by preheating to 400 degrees Fahrenheit.

2. Combine broccoli florets, olive oil, and garlic in a bowl. Season with salt and pepper to taste. Toss to blend.

3. Pour it onto a greased baking pan and spread evenly.

4. Bake until florets are tender but crisp for about 15-20 minutes. When done, transfer to a serving dish. Sprinkle with lemon extract before serving.

Nutritional Value: Calories – 49; Net Carbs – 7 grams; Protein – 2.9 grams; Fat – 1.9 grams

#25 – Sheet Pan Fajitas

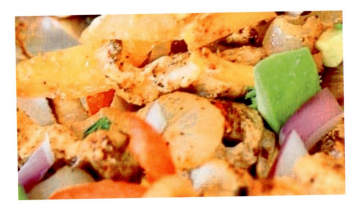

Ingredients

- 1 Red pepper (sliced)

- ¼ cup Olive oil

- ½ tsp. Garlic powder

- 1 lb. Chicken breasts (julienned)

- 1 Yellow pepper (julienned)

- 2 tsp. Chili powder

- 1 Green pepper (julienned)

- 1 Onion (julienned_

- 1 tsp. Cumin

- ½ tsp. Ground pepper

- 1 tsp. Sea salt

- A pinch of chili flakes

Directions

1. Combine chili powder, chili flakes, garlic, and cumin with oil. Season with salt and peppers

2. In another bowl, add the chicken, vegetables, and the mixture. Toss to coat evenly.

3. Pour it over a greased baking pan and spread evenly.

4. Preheat oven to 400 degrees Fahrenheit and bake chicken for 30 minutes or until cooked. Make sure that the vegetables are soft but crispy.

5. Serve in a platter with sour cream, tortillas, avocado and any of your favorite fajita toppings.

Nutritional Value: Calories – 241; Net Carbs – 6.8 grams; Protein – 16.9 grams; Fat – 16.4 grams

#26 - Skillet Green Peas

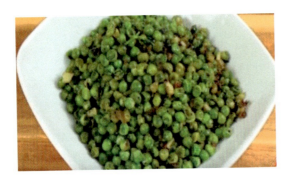

Ingredients

- 1 lb. Green beans

- 1 ½ tsp. Sesame oil

- 1 tbsp. Soy Sauce

Directions

1. Preheat a large cast-iron skillet over high-medium heat. Add the green beans and cook for 15-20 minutes, tossing continuously until it is cooked through and still crispy.

2. Serve as a side dish.

Nutritional Value: Calories – 84; Net Carbs – 16 grams; Protein – 6.1 grams; Fat – 0.2 grams

#27 - Spinach with Cream

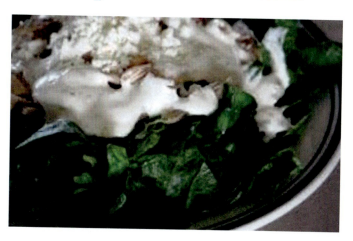

Ingredients

- 2 Bunches of Spinach (chopped)

- 1/2 cup Heavy cream

- 2 tbsp. Butter

- 1 Clove of garlic

- 1 onion (minced)

- 1 tbsp. Olive oil

- 1/4 tsp. Freshly ground nutmeg

- Freshly ground black pepper with salt to taste

Directions

1. Melt butter in a skillet over medium-high heat. Add olive oil.

2. Sauté garlic and onions for 2 minutes until soften and then add chopped spinach.

3.   Add seasonings, nutmeg, and heavy cream. Stir to mix. Cook just enough to reduce liquid by half for about 3 minutes so as not overcook spinach.

Nutritional Value: Calories – 166; Net Carbs – 4 grams; Protein – 7grams; Fat – 13 grams

#28 -Tomato Bun Tuna Melts

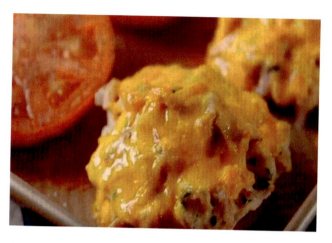

Ingredients

- 2 6-oz. Cans of tuna (drained)

- ¼ cup Mayonnaise

- ¼ Red onion (julienned)

- 1 tbsp. Dijon mustard

- Freshly ground Black pepper

- 2 cups Yellow cheddar (shredded)

- Juice extract from half lemon

- 4 Large tomatoes

- Kosher salt

Directions

2. Mix tuna, mustard, onion, mayonnaise, and parsley in a mixing bowl. Add the lemon extracted from half lemon fruit and sprinkle with salt and pepper to taste.

3. Cut tomatoes in three parts cross-wise and save the middle segment for later use.

4. Place tomatoes on a baking sheet with top and bottom face facing upwards. Spoon tuna mixture over bottom halves and place cheddar over top halves. Season with salt and pepper.

5. Broil until the bun is golden brown and the cheddar melts. This will take about 4-5 minutes of cooking.

Nutritional Value: Calories –437; Net Carbs – 3 grams; Protein – 7 grams; Fat – 44 grams

#29 – Veggie Salad -Mackerel with Egg

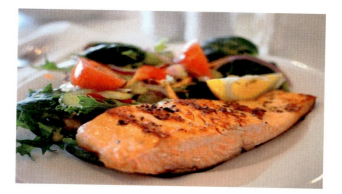

Ingredients

- 8 oz. Mackerel in tomato sauce (in the can)

- 1 Large eggs

- 2 oz. Lettuce

- ¼ cup Olive oil

- 2 tbsp. Butter

- ½ Red onion

- Salt and pepper to taste

Directions

1. Cleanse veggies and slice as desired. Chill in the refrigerator for a few hours before for a crispier vegetable salad.

2. Cook your eggs the way you want them done. You can have then sunny side up or scrambled.

3.   In a mixing bowl, add lettuce, mackerel, and slices of red onions. Season with salt and pepper and drizzle it with olive oil.

4.   Arrange your vegetable salad with mackerel together with the eggs. Serve.

Nutritional Value: Calories – 609; Net Carbs – 16.1 grams; Protein – 27.3 grams; Fat – 49.9 grams

#30 - Tomatoes with Beans and Sausage

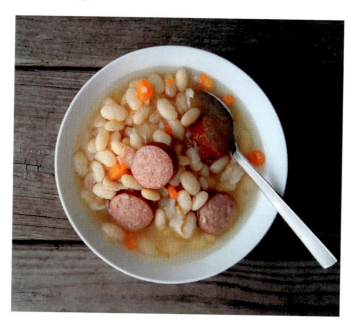

Ingredients

- 2 Italian sausages

- 1 Onion

- 2 Cloves of Garlic

- 1 tbsp. Olive oil

- 1/2 tsp. Basil (dried)

- 1/2 tsp. Oregano (dried)

- 28-oz. can Crushed tomatoes

- A pinch of Red pepper flakes

- Ground pepper (freshly cracked)

- 2 15-oz. cans of White Beans

- Sea salt to taste

Directions

- Add olive oil in a cooking pot and fry sausages in medium-low heat until brown. Once cooked, cut sausages into slices and return to pot.

- Sauté with garlic and onions until sausages become evenly browned and later transparent. While stirring, scrape the bits of sausages off the bottom of the pot. Add crushed tomatoes, add spices and seasonings.

- Meanwhile, rinse white beans with water and drain. Add beans to the pot along with chopped spinach. Stir and allow to heat through for about 10 minutes. Add salt to taste. Simmer longer to reduce the amount of liquid if you want to have a thicker consistency and serve hot with crusty bread.

Nutritional Value: Calories – 145.6; Net Carbs – 0.4 grams; Protein – 16.7 grams; Fat – 8.2 grams

Conclusion

Keto fat bombs are indeed among the most flavorful recipes that you can make if you want to enjoy delicious snacks or meal replacements. What's even better about them is that they are easy to prepare. In fact, the majority of the keto fat bomb recipes in this book can be prepared in just ten minutes.

You also have the option of making either savory or sweet fat bombs depending on what you really prefer in terms of taste. Start making fat bombs and including them in your daily routines now and you will notice their effectiveness in making you feel energized while also filling you, thereby lessening your cravings.

-- Rick Elliot

30499292R00043

Made in the USA
Lexington, KY
10 February 2019